The Intelligent MADMAN

How To Live a Healthy Life After Experiencing Mental Illness
(Schizophrenia)

PIOUS ENWEREONU

COPYRIGHT

Copyright © 2021

Pious Enwereonu

No part of this book must be copied or printed for commercial gain or profit without obtaining written permission from the author.
For permission requests, inquiries, and consultations please contact the author via any of the following media:

Email: enwereonupious402021@gmail.com

Telephone/ Whatsapp: +234 8133960831

Written by: Pious Enwereonu

TABLE OF CONTENTS

COPYRIGHT	2
DEDICATION	4
ACKNOWLEDGMENTS	5
PREFACE	6
CHAPTER ONE	10
INTERPERSONAL [RELATIONSHIP] INTELLIGENCE	10
CHAPTER TWO	30
INTRAPERSONAL [INDIVIDUAL] INTELLIGENCE	30
CHAPTER THREE	51
THE STORY OF MY MADNESS: MENTAL ILLNESS	51
[SCHIZOPHRENIA]	51
CHAPTER FOUR	65
INTUITIVE INTELLIGENCE	65
CHAPTER FIVE	70
ABSTRACT INTELLIGENCE	70
CONCLUSION	75
ABOUT THE BOOK	76
ABOUT THE AUTHOR	77

DEDICATION

This book is dedicated to Jehovah God, the epitome of wisdom, understanding, discernment, insight, and intelligence.

ACKNOWLEDGMENTS

I greatly appreciate Dr. Emmanuel CS Ojukwu, CP rtd, whose invitation to his book launch when he was the Assistant Commissioner of Police in charge of Criminal Investigation Department Imo State- rekindled my desire to be a published author.

I am deeply grateful to Dr. Vincent Egbuna Okaa, CP rtd. The former CP Force Forensic Laboratory under whose watch I worked as an AFIS [Automated Fingerprint Identification System] Operator.

With great pleasure, I acknowledge SP Lawrence Sunday Ukeme, my compassionate Commander, who grants me access to have good medical care for my illness.

Other people worthy of acknowledgment and indebtedness are my friends: Mr. Festus O.Njoku, Divine O. Mpieri, Zebulon C. Ukaegbu, Ezeah O. Linus, and Jephthah U.Ogbodo.

These men have been of immense help to me during and after each episode of my illness.

PREFACE

I define intelligence as the ability to use the knowledge of one's environment and human nature to achieve one's objective.
Most intelligent people are less likely to learn from their mistakes or take advice from others. Intellectual humility and open-mindedness are weapons to fight against what David Robson called "The intelligence trap."

So I encourage the reader to be open-minded so that he/she can gain insights and distinctions that could be applied in one's life.

I must admit that the construct called intelligence has become as broad as any other scientific discipline. No one definition fits it all because what is considered intelligent in one culture at times is different from another. And as such researchers have continued to innovate new constructs.

US cognitive scscient Steven Pinker said that "We may have trouble defining intelligence but we recognize it when we see it."

In this modern age, researchers in the field of psychology and other sister disciplines have churned out many constructs that are aimed at unraveling the nature of intelligence as a discipline.

To this end, they have propounded theories upon theories aimed at deciphering the nature of intelligence.
To achieve the goal of 'constructing a valuable society' through 'universal measurement tools', psychology researchers, and other helping professions started to innovate intelligence testing tools.

Since 1905 when French psychologist Alfred Binet devised the first intelligent test to identify slow learners in school, there have been different theories of intelligence formulated by psychologists and experts.

The following are a good number of theories formulated among others. General intelligence was formulated by Charles Spearman in 1904. He opined that intelligence is a general mental ability that underlies all intellectual capabilities.

Primary and mental ability was formulated by Louis L. Thurstone in 1938. His theory of intelligence consisted of seven independent abilities: (1) verbal comprehension (2) verbal fluency (3) number or arithmetic ability (4) memory (5) executive speed (6) inductive reasoning and (7) spatial visualization.

After Thurstone came Raymond B. Cattle and John Horn who jointly propounded the theory of fluid intelligence and crystallized intelligence in 1966. In their view, fluid intelligence is a biologically-based capacity for reasoning and memory. Crystallized intelligence is knowledge acquired through experience and learning.

Psychologist Howard Gardner proposed the multiple intelligence theory in 1983 which included seven separate abilities: They are (1) linguistic intelligence (2) musical intelligence (3) logical-mathematical intelligence (4) spatial intelligence (5) bodily-kinesthetic intelligence (6) interpersonal intelligence (7) intrapersonal intelligence and (8) naturalistic intelligence which he added after amending his theory in the 1990s.

Psychologist Robert Sternberg, believing that intelligence involves more than the foregoing, proposed a triarchic theory of intelligence. In it he theorized that intelligence consists of three major parts namely:(1) analytical intelligence -skills in reasoning and processing information. (2) creative intelligence -skill in using past experiences to achieve the insight and dealing with new situations. (3) Practical intelligence- skill in everyday living and in adapting to life's demands.

In this book, I will excerpt the titles of the first two chapters from Howard Gardner's Interpersonal and intrapersonal intelligence. This book is written for the millions of individuals who are suffering from mental illness [schizophrenia]

The caregivers of those who are suffering from schizophrenia and those who live a healthy life but who wants to know what it is like to experience madness- schizophrenia.

The cause of schizophrenia is not known. But scientists believe that there are factors that are probable causes of the illness. Knowledge of these factors will help the reader to have an idea of the nature of the illness.

While the reader will find most of the author's life experiences in chapter 3-the story of my madness, the reader is also encouraged to delve into chapters 1 and 2 which deals with relationships and individual intelligence.

Chapter 1 shows how a lack of knowledge of how to relate well with other people in one's life and environment is one contributing factor to relationship problems.

Chapter 2 deals with belief systems that cause an individual to have low self-esteem, dwelling in negative self-talk that contributes to a lack of peace of mind and maladaptive behaviors.

Chapters 4 and 5 introduce the reader to other ways of thinking that enhance creativity and intellectual growth.

CORPOREAL [PHYSICAL] INTELLIGENCE

" When I was small and easily wounded books we are my carapace. If I were recalled to my hurt in the middle of a book they somehow mattered less. My Corporeal life was slight the dazzling one in my head [and] was what really mattered. Returning to books was coming home." -Lauren Groff.

CHAPTER ONE

INTERPERSONAL [RELATIONSHIP] INTELLIGENCE

This is the ability to use knowledge of human nature to achieve peaceful and harmonious coexistence through effective and empathic communication.

According to Howard Gardner, interpersonal intelligence is the ability to understand other people, what motivates them, how they work, and how to work cooperatively with them. He further stated that it includes abilities to discern and respond accordingly to the moods, temperaments, motivations, and desires of other people. "The ability to handle people well is more valuable than all other leadership and management traits put together." John D. Rockefeller.

You probably already know that managing or leading humans is considered one of the most difficult things in life by many. To that end, how would you treat the knowledge of effective interpersonal relation. No doubt you may appreciate it for the reason that you would like to enjoy personal peace of mind- which mainly comes from being at peace with others.

Humans are dynamic creatures. To relate effectively with them you need to adapt consistently to their moods, temperaments, motivations, and desires. This adaptation does not mean that you have to completely abandon your moods, temperaments, motivations, and desires. It means being able to integrate your own with that of others and even allowing people to realize their objective temporarily before yours. Philippians 2:4.

"What do we live for if not to make the world less difficult for each other." -George Eliot once wrote.
Some may not like the idea of pleasing others even before themselves because of selfish human nature. And you probably already know that selfishness is a major cause of quarreling in human relationships.

"The experienced analyst of human character judges people not by their words but by the feeling or lack of feeling they unconsciously impart with their words." -Andrew Carnegie, Rich industrialist.
Cultivating interpersonal intelligence calls for mastering the ability to discern the feelings imparted into words 'unconsciously.'

Granted it is very difficult to understand what is going on in another person's unconscious or subconscious mind when one is not schooled in the psychological or psychiatric disciplines. Psychologists, psychiatrists, and neuroscientists are only beginning to decipher the fringes of the recesses of man's mind. To enable the reader to understand what it is like to be another person, we will use the four human temperaments of medieval physiology.

TEMPERAMENTS
There are four humor [ous] temperaments. They are the melancholy [melancholic],phlegmatic, Sanguine, and Choleric. See Proverbs chapter 30:11-14.

"If a Sanguine person enters warm and enthusiastic, the phlegmatic person becomes cold as ice. Melancholy [melancholic] comes along pessimistically lamenting the miseries of the world, the phlegmatic become more optimistic than ever and teases them beyond endurance. If a choleric enters the room brimful with plans and projects, it is an exquisite pleasure for the phlegmatic to throw cold water on their enthusiasm, and with their level-headedness and keen understanding it is an easy matter for them to point out the weaknesses of the choleric's proposition." Dr. Ole Khristian Hallesby.

Despite whatever temperament you may have due to heredity it is instructive to note that God's active force or holy spirit can energize you to cultivate qualities that are essential for harmonious coexistence with others. See Galatians chapter 5 verses 22 and 23.
Unfortunately, the Holy Spirit cannot operate on those who do not obey and worship God according to his terms. See John 4:23 24; Proverbs 28:9; Luke 11:13. The habit of reading God's word and accepting help for an accurate understanding of its teachings is a stepping-stone to everlasting benefits. See John 17:3 Psalms 25:14.

A truly intimate relationship with the true God Jehovah has a positive effect on a person's relationship with others notwithstanding his or her inherent temperament. The existence of temperaments creates room for a variety of traits in society. Henry Van Dyke said that "In the progress of personality first comes a declaration of independence than a recognition of interdependence."

Lack of knowledge of the existence of temperaments contributes to most frictions in relationships. The realization that one's behavior tends to resemble attributes of a given temperament, should not make a person feel that he is destined to a life with fixed sets of unchangeable behavioral traits. If an individual makes an examination of his personality and finds out that he has some flaws that hinder interdependence, he should endeavor to put on a new personality that contributes to peaceful coexistence. See Ephesians 4:24.

A philosopher once said that an unexamined life is not worth living. In an interdependent world, individual self-examination on the effect of one's behavior on others is essential but self-examination to the point of merciless introspection is counterproductive. Unfortunately, that is what the melancholic temperament does.

Dr. Ole Khristian Hallesby, in his book, Temperament and the Christian Faith explained the life of a melancholic. He that a melancholic "is surely more self-centered than any of the other temperaments. He is inclined to that kind of self-examination, that kind of self-contemplation that paralyzes his Will and energy. He is always dissecting his mental conditions, taking off layer after layer as an onion is peeled, until there is nothing direct and artless left in his life; there is only his everlasting self-examination. This self-examination is not only unfortunate; it is harmful.

Melancholy usually drifts into morbid mental conditions. They are also unduly concerned about their physical condition. Everything that touches a melancholic is of prime importance to him, hence no other type can so easily become a hypochondriac." The purpose of self-examination is usually to see that one's actions are in tandem with one's goals, values, and purpose of existence. When there is dissonance, the necessary thing to do is to take action to correct such attitudes that are both inimical to one's peace of mind and counterproductive in peaceful relations with others. Sadly egotism hinders such necessary corrective action.

"Egotists have a tough time in marriage. Their interests tend to be in outside activities, such as jobs and hobbies, rather than in the home. This doesn't mean that they don't care about the marriage, but rather that they derive more fulfillment from their accomplishments than from relationships... To them, anyone who does not fit with their plans is a source of irritation. The egotist has several fears which influence his lack of trust in people. He fears that he is not as significant as he would like to believe. And he greatly fears being controlled by other people. To him, being vulnerable will be used against him, so he resists closeness even though in many cases, he truly desires it.

He cannot imagine divulging his future feelings, thoughts, and goals to another person. Even though his fears are misguided, it is very difficult to convince him otherwise. The only person he ends up trusting is himself."-Dr. David Field, in his book Marriage Personalities.

RELATIONSHIPS
Studies have shown that sustaining positive relationships are one of the known factors that contribute to happiness in life. Therefore, if you feel unhappy most of your life, check how well you relate with people and you may be surprised in your finding if that check is honest self-examination.

Dr. S.I. McMillen said that he could "recall how many times...[he] had to make house calls on patients when...[he] was not feeling well...[him]self .... [He] found that the stress of making the trip often cured... [him] of...[his] minor aches and pains. However, if...[he] made the trip in the Spirit of antagonism...[his] faulty reaction might have put...[him] in the hospital for a week. Is it not a remarkable feat that our stress reaction determines whether stress is going to kill us or make us sick?

Here is an important key to longer and happier living. We hold the key a land can decide whether [the] stress [encountered during interactions with fellow humans] is going to work for us or against us."

It is improbable to have inner peace of mind without being at peace with others because we are all created to connect.
"The desire for connection is a basic human need. It is so powerful that when people don't feel connected, they're far more likely to develop addictions. The pain of empty relationships is so great that they go looking for some way to medicate the hollow feeling, to cover it over with some numbing pleasure."- Psychologist Gary Smalley.

Evolutionary theory has done more harm than good to humanity. By treating fellow humans as subhumans or as animals, the evolutionary mindset accentuates the downgrading of equal basic human needs through its social Darwinism.
This is because it is "Within the context of relationship can the deepest needs of human personality be met. People everywhere long for intimate relationships. We all need to be close to someone. Make no apology for your strong desire to be intimate with someone; it is neither sinful nor selfish. Don't ignore the need by preoccupying yourself with peripheral satisfactions such as social achievement or acquiring knowledge. Neglecting your longing for a relationship by claiming to be above it is as foolish as pretending you can live without food.

Our need for a relationship is real and it is there by God's design."-Larry Crabb, in his book: The Marriage Builder.

While it is not 'sinful' to have an 'intimate relationship with another human of the opposite sex when married, it is sinful to have an intimate relationship with a person of the opposite sex to the point of sex when not married or with the same sex to the point of sex whether married or not. See Hebrews 13:4;Romans 1:26,27.

It is a human need to have the so-called platonic friendship but it is sinful to disregard God's moral laws on the platitude of relationships. See Ist Corinthians 6:9 and 10.
To have a successful relationship each party should know that "silence will destroy a relationship quicker than any other methods." -Psychologist Bob Philip advised.

Therefore, respond to the need for connection by getting connected to the person who wants to fill that need. Granted there are times when one may be too busy to respond to messages, calls, or other demands of loved ones, friends, and acquaintances. The respite is to reciprocate as soon as one is unhindered. The fact is "A blessed thing it is for any man or woman to have a friend, one human soul whom we can trust utterly, who knows the best and worst of us, and who loves us despite all our faults." - Charles Kingsley. See Proverbs 17:17.

Have friends only with those who have good values and morals because bad friends corrupt good morals. See Proverbs 13:20.
It is in true friendship or relationship that one's confidence is entrusted because true friends can keep one's secret more than physical relations. See Proverbs 18:24.

Furthermore "In poverty, and other misfortunes of life, true friends are a sure refuge. The young they keep out of mischief, to the old they are a comfort and aid in their weakness and those in

the prime of life they incite to noble deeds."-Aristotle.
As a 'friend', I intend to 'incite you to "noble deeds" that are enshrined in God's word the Bible [Psalms 1:1- 3] but if you use any of the knowledge in this book to engage in ignoble 'deeds' be sure to bear the consequences.
If I unknowingly offended you by the preceding words what should you do?
You should "Keep a fair-sized cemetery in your backyard; in which to bury the faults of your friends." -Henry Ward Beecher advised.
I am not a friend of the world alienated from the life that belongs to God. (James 4:4).
Why then did you write this book? I wrote it because of this fact: "Genuine friends encourage and challenge us to live out our best...." -Dan Reiland wrote.

So to earn my friendship you ought to be ready to always 'live out your best by using your life to worship the true God Jehovah who created you. See Revelation 4:11.
For "If the first law of friendship is that it has to be cultivated, the second law is to be indulgent when the first law has been neglected."-Voltaire.

To be indulgent with you in this friendship of ours, I would like to let you know that the name of my God is Jehovah. Jehovah is the name of God as revealed in the Bible. He holds me accountable for my actions in life. See Ecclesiastes chapter 12 verses 13 and 14.
He is my friend forever. See Psalms 25:14. He rewards me for worshiping him. See Hebrews 11:6.

Does it surprise you that I said that God is my friend, best friend for that matter? It shouldn't because in the Bible the patriarch

Abraham was called God's friend at James 2:23. So if Abraham could be God's friend you too can. This can be done if you can exercise faith in him and be loyal to him. God will also be loyal to you according to Psalms 18:25.

Apart from God, I also have another special friend in the person of my Lord Jesus Christ.
He gave his life for me. See John 3:16; Galatians 2:20. And it is through him that I have the privilege to form a friendship with God. See John 15:13,14; 14:6.

I also have several human friends and I would like to mention three of these who have been of great benefit to me, especially during my madness or mental illness. They are brothers Festus O. Njoku, Zebulon C. Ukaegbu, and Jephthah U. Ogbodo. Sometimes, when I am experiencing the symptoms of my mental illness [schizophrenia] even if it is midnight, I would call them with my phone and they would ask me questions like: Have you taken your drugs? Have you eaten? My answer to the questions would give them a clue as to the next kind of help they would render -even though they are not psychologists or psychiatrists. If I have not taken my drugs because it has finished and I didn't have money to buy them at that material time, they will make arrangements for me to get my drug and resume taking it.

I am grateful to God for having these friends in my life. If you are a sufferer of mental illness especially schizophrenia, have good social support. What social support means is your relatives, friends, and acquaintances who are around you, encouraging you.

Listen to their advice that is not against your doctor's treatment regimen. Some of the symptoms of schizophrenia include the belief that others are persecuting you whether it is real or imagined. Remember that your relatives and close friends mean well to you. At times because of the nature of the illness, your mind may deceive you into thinking that your relatives or friends are your enemies. Reject that thought. In chapter 3 of this book, you will know why you have such thoughts. Tell them how lucky you are to have them as your relatives or friends. Because at times owing to the challenge of caring for you, they may become overwhelmed with anxieties.

Why am I telling you all this? The reason is that "The most I can do for my friend is simply to be his friend." Henry David Thoreau.
What if a friend does not appreciate friendly advice?
If he or she doesn't want you to be his or her friend anymore, remember that "You can make more friends in two months by becoming interested in other people than you can in two years by trying to get other people interested in you." -Dale Carnegie.

A person who is easily interested in people with an enthusiastic Sanguine temperament can make new friends. What if a person's personality makes it difficult to find new friends. He can first unlearn the habits that are hampering his easy bonding with people.
It is even counterproductive to have plenty of friends without solid close friends that could stay the test of time. Before venturing into making more friends, my advice as a friend is that you should "Look carefully at the closest associations in your life, for that is the direction you are heading."Kevin Eikenberry. See Ist Corinthians 15:33.

Whether you are young or old you need friendship. Children also need it. That is why self-esteem is high in families where children see their parents as their friends. What happens when the reverse is the case? Then pay attention to Neil Anderson author of Victory over Darkness. He wrote that "Studies have shown that, in the average home, for every positive statement a child receives [ten] 10 negative statements. The school environment is only slightly better, students hear seven negative statements from their teachers for every one positive statement. No wonder so many children are growing up feeling that they are losers. Parents and teachers are conveying that perception every day in how they talk to their children. These studies go on to point out that it takes four positive statements to negate the effect of one negative statement."

Parents make your children your friends by setting standards of good behavior for them. Implement the standards of discipline. Associate with them as friends do. Teach them good behavior by your actions. Remember they learn more through feelings than through reasoning.
Furthermore "Children will not remember you for the material things you provided but for feeling that you cherished them."- Richard L. Evans.

Parents being friends of their children does not mean spoiling them, but being permissive will. Socrates corroborated this point when he said that "Those who provide much wealth for their children but neglect to improve them in virtue do like those who feed their horses high but never trained them to be useful."

You probably already know that when children are properly trained, one day they will become responsible adults. A responsible single adult who is in an intimate relationship with a member of the opposite sex is probably contemplating...

MARRIAGE

Historically, marriage is a legal or formal union between a man and a woman in a personal relationship.

Furthermore, the union is meant to be permanent. It was not intended to be a playground for trial and error as seen in most cultures where the sentence reads, "And they lived happily ever after is one of the tragic sentences in literature. Is tragic because it is a falsehood. It is a myth that has led generations to expect something from a marriage that is not possible."-Joshua Lieberman. Romantic movies and novels are filled with fairy tales on marriage. These tales drive intending couples to nurture inane expectations that in most cases do not exist in married life. "Mutual enthusiasm, therefore, is usually the basis of marriage and woe unto the party to the marriage who usually allows that enthusiasm to wane afterward. We speak of the relationship as love, but what is love but mutual enthusiasm of two people over each other." -Andrew Carnegie.

For a marriage relationship to succeed, the married couple needs to work as a team. Marriage is an institution. In it, you will see workers, management, and customers transacting business daily.

In this institution, parents serve as management. Their work is to oversee the workers or staff - which is the children if childbearing had resulted, if not, they attend to the customers-the public or society. It is trite knowledge that an institution or organization is managed by the executives which are simply referred to as the management. What is the centerpiece of management? Leadership experts Warren Bennis and Burt Nanus answered that what they "have found is that the higher the rank the more interpersonal and human the undertaking. Our top executives spend roughly 90% of the time with others and virtually the same amount of time concerned with the messiness of people's problems."

So it is with marriage. Throughout the marriage, married couples are concerned with the messiness of people, the problem of raising their children into responsible adults, if they have children, or the problem of attending to the customers of the institution that is the public, if they do not have children.

If you are single but contemplating marriage, are you prepared to manage this institution called marriage? If you are not, please read carefully: "You have to live with yourself at least reasonably well before you are to leave with a mate. There must be certain self-esteem before you can expect that other people will value you highly."-Theodor Reik advised.

After self-examination and delegation of one's ability and willingness to undertake the business called marriage, the next thing to do is to prepare for the recruitment of workers or staff which is children. That is why a child psychiatrist Dr. Stanley Greenspan wrote that
"Emotional development and interactions form the foundation for all children's learning -especially in the first five years of life. During these years, children abstract from their emotional experiences constantly to learn even the most basic concepts."

Parents who do not have emotional maturity cannot be able to manage their emotional ups and downs and as such endanger the emotional well-being of their children. This lack of maturity has a great impact on the life of children. This fact is well attested to in cases of sadomasochistic and sadistic actions in some adults. When couples are ill-prepared for marriage, child-rearing becomes a venture of trial-and-error. How did they come into this state of affairs? It was as a result of prior...

ROMANTIC FANTASY

Romance novels and movies propagate the fantasy that passionate relationships lead to permanent union.
That is why "When two people are under the influence of the most violent, most insane, most delusive, and most transient of passions, they are required to swear that they will remain in that excited, abnormal, and exhaustive condition continuously until death do them part."-George Bernard Shaw.

Unprepared marriages are filled with passion instead of maturity. The illusion of couples who enter into marriage without emotional maturity is that marriage is only a legitimate institution where they can quench their passion for sex.

Granted, sex within marriage between persons of the opposite sex is the only platform that has divine approval, (Proverbs 5:15-20;1 Corinthians 7:2) but there is more to marriage than sex. See 1Corinthians 7:4,5; Ephesians 5:22-25 ,28 ,29.

Men and women do not think alike on issues. This is why married people must consider the views of their mate when a problem arises. One woman who has passed menopause once said that she would talk matters over with her husband, and after his sympathetic understanding, she would see that the problems weren't as big as her anxious state of mind made them. See 1Peter 3:7.

To manage an institution effectively, you must acquire managerial skills. John Ruskin once said that "When love and skill work together expect a masterpiece."
Lack of consideration and understanding is one of the factors that lead to marriage disintegration -separation or divorce.
Lack of proper management of an institution is a reason why an

institution goes bankrupt within a few years of doing business.

Business Management is similar to relationship management. So "If I am attached to another person because I cannot stand on my own two feet, he or she may be a lifesaver, but the relationship is not one of love." -Erich Fromm.
How can one know a premarital relationship that is 'of love' from that of romantic fantasy?

You should know that "Young Love Is a flame; very pretty, very hot and fierce, but still only light and flickering. The love of the older and disciplined heart is as coals, deep-burning, unquenchable." -Henry Ward Beecher wrote.

Granted, studies have shown that the first nine months to one year of a premarital the relationship is very hot as a flame, you can still understand its presence or absence after the dissipation of that passionate fire.

Leo Tolstoy told us the reason when he said that "There are as many minds as there are heads, so there are as many kinds of love as there are hearts."

So ladies and gentlemen, when you hear the words: "I love you" ask for specificity.
Why? Because research has proven that men, more than women, tend to express such words. Which type of love does the speaker mean? Is it agape, platonic, erotic, filial?
Please can you figure out which type the following expression belongs to? "I love thee to the depth and breadth and height my soul can reach." -Elizabeth Barrett Browning. No doubt you understand the point. If you are an unmarried woman, how can you know for sure that this man is not infatuated with you?

Katherine Anne Porter answered the question when she wrote that "Love must be learned and learned again and again." She added that "There is no end to it." If he loves you, he will continue to love you no matter what, except if you people are incompatible. 1st Corinthians chapter 13 verses 4-8 defines what true love is.

Read it and practice it to derive the most benefit.
What if you are an unmarried man seeking a good marriage mate? Know this fact by Elizabeth Stoddard, "A woman despises a Man for Loving her unless she returns his love."
Unmarried men should know that women do not think the same way as they do. They are more emotional than men. So even if you receive a quick positive reply to your proposition, you probably already know now that she needs considerable time to think properly about your proposal or vice versa.

Why did I give the above advice? It is because "Half of the secret of getting along with people is consideration of their views, the other half is tolerance in one's view."-Daniel Frohman.

GENUINE LOVE
Agape is a word that represents what genuine love involves. It is love that is motivated by knowledge of God, his principles and standards. One who has this love can distinguish between platonic and erotic love.

Antoine De Saint-Exupery once said that "True love is inextinguishable: the more you give, the more you have. And if you go to draw at the true fountainhead, the more water you draw, the more abundant its flow."
Love is the very embodiment of the true God Jehovah. It was this quality that motivated him to bring all creation into existence. See Ist John 4:8: Revelation 4:11.

Our ability to love our neighbors, friends, and enemies is a true reflection of the possession of this sterling attribute. See Matthew 22:37-40; 5:44-45.

The love of God and neighbor is an active form of love. Psychiatrist Erik Fromm corroborated this line of thought when he said that "Love is an active power in man [kind]; a power which breaks through the walls which separate man from his fellow men, which unites him with others; love makes him overcome the sense of isolation and separateness, yet it permits him to be himself to retain his integrity. Envy, jealousy, ambition, any kind of greed are passions; love is an action, the practice of a human power, which can be practiced only in freedom and never as the result of a compulsion."

When we exhibit genuine love for another human, we heal ourselves both spiritually and physically because Love is a divine quality that caused our very existence. Joseph Conrad once wrote that it is "only in man's imagination does every truth find an effective and undeniable existence. Imagination, not invention, is the supreme master of the art, as of life."

It is an "undeniable" fact "of life" that in the family genuine love makes a husband and wife cooperate in the running of the institution under the empathic direction of the chief executive officer- the husband. See Ist Corinthians 11:3.

C.S. Lewis gives us a description of what filial love is when he said that he and his wife "feasted on love; every mode of it, solemn and merry, romantic, and realistic. Sometimes as dramatic as a thunderstorm, sometimes comfortable and unemphatic as putting on your soft slippers.

She was my pupil and my teacher, my subject and my sovereign, my trusty [trusted] comrade, friend, shipmate, a fellow soldier.

My mistress but at the same time all that any man has ever been to me."

That is it. Husbands, exercise your God-given headship with humility and love in your family. Wives, be submissive and empowering compliments of your husbands.
Communicate always to plan for marital success and join resources to solve any problem that ensues in your union because "marriage is one long conversation chequered by
disputes [owing to human imperfection]."-Robert Louis Stevenson. 1Corinthians 7:28.
In addition to love and communication, another quality is essential for lasting marital union. That quality is...

TRUST
What is it? It is a belief that what a person is telling you is true and seeking no further proof
We can learn some lessons on trust from the former US Secretary of State Henry L. Simpson. He said that "The chief lesson I have learned in a long life is that the only way you can make a man trustworthy is by trusting him, and the surest way to make him untrustworthy is to distrust him and show your distrust."

If you want to be trusted, trust another human by always telling him the truth. This does not mean divulging the confidence of others to those who are not entitled to it. If you are trustworthy, people will entrust you with their confidences, their cares, and secrets that others who might be close to them do not know. Can you imagine the effect of letting the cat out of the bag?
Disintegrated relationships can be traced to untrustworthiness. Socrates advised that if you want to marry "By all means marry; if you get a good wife, you will become happy. If you get a bad one you will become a philosopher."

The author of this book has clarified how a healthy relationship throughout marriage or singleness could be sustained.

Therefore, he does not subscribe to the cynical perception of marriage institutions that accentuate its aversion and subsequent substitution with promiscuous relationships. If one cannot maintain faithfulness towards one's marriage mate can he/she maintain faithfulness in other human relationships?

Could lack knowledge of what a marriage mate wants and inability to satisfy such need be the reason for disenchantment and subsequent rampant infidelity?
Using human wisdom to manage an institution instituted by God is the bane of acrimonies seen in this institution called marriage.See Genesis 1:27 ,28; 2:22-24; Isaiah 48:17,18.
It is instructive to note that Sigmund Freud, one of the noted mind scientists could not even decipher what a woman wants.

The Holy bible stated unequivocally and simply the want of a woman amongst other things: "Husbands should love their wives as their bodies. A man who loves his wife loves himself. For no one ever hated his own body, but he feeds and cherishes it." - Ephesians 5:28,29.

Dave Barry concurred with the above biblical line of thought when he said that "What women want
To be loved, to be listened to,
To be desired, to be respected,
To be needed, to be trusted, and sometimes, just to be held.
What men want, Tickets for the world series."

Having known what a woman wants will equip a man to know how to treat a woman.

This is irrespective of whether a man is married or not.

For men who are unmarried but are contemplating marriage, this foreknowledge will help you to handle your relationship with decorum -until marriage issues.

To the married men, continue to use the above biblical and relevant secular quotes to enhance the stability of your marriage. This also applies to women. If you have a solid marital relationship there would be no room for contemplating divorce when faced with challenges in marriage.

When the marriage relationship is stable "There may be nothing more important in a marriage than a determination that it should persist. With such a determination, individuals force themselves to adjust and accept situations which otherwise seem sufficient grounds for a breakup." -Dr. Alfred Kinsey advised. See Matthew 19: 9; Hebrews 13:4; Malachi 2:14-16.

CHAPTER TWO

INTRAPERSONAL [INDIVIDUAL] INTELLIGENCE

This is an ability to connect to oneself through an open-minded reflection on one's conscious and subconscious processes.

According to Howard Gardner the author of Frames of Mind "it is a capacity to form an accurate, veridical model of oneself and to be able to use that model to operate effectively in life."
Gardner further defined intrapersonal intelligence as the capacity to assess one's feelings and the ability to discriminate among them and draw upon them to guide behavior
Those who excel in the ability, manifest self-esteem, self-acceptance, and confidence without confusing the same with pride.

Phil McGraw concurred with this line of thought when he wrote, "I always say that the most important relationship you will ever have is with yourself.
You've got to be your own best friend first."
Those who do not possess this ability are at the mercy of their whims and caprices and often live in fool's paradise as a subterfuge to ameliorate their internal dissonance.
Intrapersonal intelligence is essential in life because of the reason that "He who knows much about others may be learned but he who understands himself is more intelligent. He who controls others may be powerful, but he who has mastered himself is mightier still."- Lao Tsu, Tao The King.

Knowledge of intrapersonal intelligence is an antidote to low self-esteem which results from demeaning self-conception orchestrated by comparing one's worth with external references.

"When I suspect the problem, I ask a person to tell me what he likes about himself. He is usually very uncomfortable; it would be much simpler if you could tell me what he does not like. His worth and values are not based upon internal personal worth but on his external performance. He may be very successful in [work,] business, or sports, but it isn't enough. He feels he has to be perfect to make up for his internally felt shortcomings." -Dr. David Field.

SELF ESTEEM

Self-esteem involves recognition and expression of one's unique talents and learning abilities without arrogance.
"If you develop your talents they will make way for you."-James Rohn once said
Those who seem to have self-esteem developed it. It was a latent disposition inherent in all humans. Why then do some have low self-esteem? Low self-esteem is another word for undeveloped self-esteem. Self-esteem is undeveloped and as such becomes low in a person when the person's conception of worth is fuelled by preconceived notions of inadequacy learned either from childhood or adulthood in an inhibitory environment.

Andrew Carnegie a rich industrialist once said that "The mental attitude of people leaves its permanent influence on the very atmosphere of their environment."

Low self-esteem is a "mental attitude" learned from one's "environment" at any stage of life. It could be learned from home, school, place of worship, business, or workplace.
Those who think that they are low in self-esteem or who feel that

they are not good enough in anything should heed this advice from Harry Emerson Fosdick: "Reduce to a minimum the things that mortify you. To be ugly, to lack desired ability, to be economically restricted, such things are limitations, but if they become humiliations it is because inwardly you make them so."

That is exactly what people with self-esteem do. They accept themselves for who they are but never allow that to go into their head.
"Truly great men and women are never
terrifying. Their humility puts you at ease."- Elizabeth Goudge. See Proverbs 15:33;29:23.

Because they are humble in heart, those who possess genuine self-esteem do not follow the crowd of people in any discipline of the life of which they might be proud.
Henry David Thoreau collaborated with this line of thought when he said that "If a man does not keep pace with his companions, perhaps, it is because he hears a different drummer. Let him step to the music which he hears, however, measured and far away."

What is that "different drummer" which a person with self-esteem hears?
Kenneth Hilderbrand answers: "Strong lives are motivated by dynamic purposes." Those who have "dynamic purposes" are those who have self-esteem. The benefits of self-esteem are that it will enable you to craft your vision and mission in life. You will not be adrift in life.

You will have a sense of purpose in life that continues to motivate you to move forward towards the attainment of your purpose of existence.

PITFALLS TO SELF ESTEEM

Avoid overconfident self-esteem for it undermines true Godliness [Proverbs 14:16]

Those who have low self-esteem from childhood might have had this mental attitude as a result of ignorant parental scripting during their nurture; those who have it in later life came to the state owing to environmental conditioning or peer influences. People in this mental state should realize that humans are dynamic creatures. So why limit oneself with that static frame of mind?

Low self-esteem or feeling of inadequacy can come when you set rigid goals that become unachievable. It can also be deduced in the habit of passing the buck when one's envisaged outcome proved abortive.

When this happens, the result would be a blame game. And does blaming others solve your problem? No. Why not? Because "All blame is a waste of time. No matter how much fault you find with another, and regardless of how much you blame him, it will not change you." - Wayne Dyer

When people use excuses as a strategy to obscure this mental attitude, the only unconscious leverage they have is to wallow in vainglorious gruff to appear important before people.

When parents fail to instill self-esteem in their children, they become low in self-esteem and easy prey to others who have high self-esteem but bad values.

This is one of the factors that lead to bad associations. One who sees himself or feels low in esteem is not the same as one who is humble and modest. A humble or modest person has self-esteem but never allows it to go into his head. My lord Jesus Christ of Nazareth and Moses the leader of ancient nation of Isreal are good examples of people with both humility and self-esteem.

Being humble or modest or having self-esteem does not presuppose that the possessor is a coward, for if it is so, the above examples would be irrelevant. This boils down to the conclusion: Low self-esteem may be a predisposing factor for cowardice. Can one with low self-esteem be able to change his or her condition?

"In reality, change is not an option. It is an ongoing, lifelong daily experience. How we change is our only option. Change begins by choosing, and choosing creates more change."-Bob Phillips, Psychologist.

To change a particular mental attitude that is ingrained calls for open-mindedness. And to be open-minded a person would have to adopt a kind of thinking that is popularly called...

POSITIVE THINKING

This is a thinking strategy that enhances the leverage of extrapolatory thinking.

Extrapolatory thinking is the act of using present positive or negative estimates of events to infer the future positive or negative outcome of such events. I'll dedicate a whole chapter on the subject of extrapolatory thinking in my future book. Positive thinking is a thinking method in which one adopts to withstand an adverse situation that seems unbearable and insurmountable when faced with a negative mindset.

"The better things of Life always go to men who form the habit of organized thinking...

Thinking constructively is one responsibility that no one can delegate to another. It is an individual responsibility ."- Andrew Carnegie.

It is your responsibility to engage in organized thinking to surmount challenges that beset you.

Whether you believe in positive thinking or not it does not matter.

What matters is that you have the responsibility to organize your thinking. If you fail to, your subconscious will start to engage in negative thinking and negative thinking leads to negative actions unless it is interrupted by positive thinking which leads an individual into positive action.

In most cases, negative thinking is leverage of negative past experiences.

That is why Collin Powell said that "None of us can change yesterdays, but all of us can change our tomorrow."

AUTOSUGGESTION [SELF-TALK]

Is "a process that makes you believe sth [something] or act in a particular way according to ideas that come from within yourself without you realizing it" -Oxford Advanced Learner's Dictionary. The 6th edition.

Autosuggestion is nothing but accumulated self-talk and thought projected to the conscious mind by the subconscious mind without the knowledge of an individual.

"There is no factor more decisive in one's psychological development and motivation than the estimate [or assessment] one passes on himself." -Nathaniel Brandon, author of The Seven Pillars of Self-esteem.

An individual may believe or act on internally generated ideas with a decisive gusto. On the false premise that it is an intuition without knowing in reality that such an internally generated Idea is an auto-suggestion. Internally-generated intuition is affected by auto-suggestion while the external is affected by Abstract-Cosmic-Magnetism.

See the chapter on intuition and abstract intelligence for the meaning of Abstract-Cosmic-Magnetism.

So, how do you talk to yourself? Do tell yourself positive words or do you choose negative words to inundate yourself? Eleanor Roosevelt told us what happens to us as a result of our choice of words when she said that "In the long run we shape our lives, the choices we make are ultimately our responsibility."

I happened to encounter a young man who is a government employee but who was made fun of by his colleagues as being slightly crazy. I was startled to hear the young man in my presence say: "My brain is not correct." When he made several mistakes in writing practice that his most senior colleague set for him as a task. I was a bit annoyed by him. I asked him, Why did you say such a thing to yourself? Is this how you have been talking to yourself for a long time? He admitted that whenever he makes mistake his master usually calls him names to the extent that he becomes downhearted and therefore gives in by accepting his negative words to save face. See Ecclesiastes 7:7.

NEGATIVE AUTOSUGGESTION
Preoccupation with negative thinking often leads to negative talking. Negative self-talk is inimical to the mental well-being of the individual without his knowledge of it. Negative autosuggestion is the same as negative self-talk. Examples are: "Why are things so always difficult for me? What have I done to people that makes all of them dislike me or why do people always hate me?

Is there any consequence of negative autosuggestion? Yes, there is, "The fundamental trouble with these people is that they are not always careful to draw the line of demarcation between self-examination and introspection. We all agree that we shall examine ourselves, but we also agree that introspection and morbidity are bad. But what is the difference between examining oneself and becoming introspective? I suggest that we cross the line from self-examination to introspection when, in a sense, we do nothing but examine ourselves, and when such self-examination becomes the main and chief end in our life."- Dr. Martyn Lloyd Jones, in his book Spiritual Depression.

The main purpose of self-examination is to find where and how a person's behavior is in discordance with his beliefs and values and to make necessary readjustments needed to live a satisfying life - which is a life that is in agreement with God's will.
"Life without true godly devotion is inane and devoid of genuine satisfaction and meaning." -Pious Enwereonu.

After correcting the young man who reactively accepted that his brain was not correct by telling him to say: my brain is correct repeatedly, the young man did so and the result was that he got the last written test correct by himself.

"The subconscious mind responds always to the dominating thoughts in one's mind. Moreover, it gets into the habit of acting quickly on the thoughts which are repeated most often." -Andrew Carnegie.

Because of what I witnessed in the presence of the young man, and his master, I got closer to him after his elder sister granted me access to study with him. I found out later that this young man has for a long time inundated himself with negative autosuggestion and that I have had a great effect on his life. His constant negative self-talk has helped him not only to become depressive but also dyslexic. "If defeat is accepted as permanent instead of being regarded as a mere stimulant to greater action, the subconscious mind acts accordingly and makes it permanent." -Andrew Carnegie advised.

Can a person whose life is enamored with negative autosuggestion be abought to change into positive autosuggestion?

Andrew Carnegie answered the question when he said that "Any state of mind, whether positive or negative, becomes a habit the moment it begins to dominate the mind."

POSITIVE AUTOSUGGESTION

"Our human brains are programmed much like a computer. ... Unlike computers, however, humans develop the habit of programming their minds to be either mostly
negative or mostly positive."-Dr Wallis

The self- suggestions or "programming" that is most dominant in a person's life explains which "habit" pattern would influence his life the most.

Auto-suggestion, self-talk, self-programming, or self-suggestion means the same thing.

We have just considered the effect that negative auto-suggestion brings to one's mind. The effect of positive or negative self-talk is realized in the face of challenging circumstances. That was what Kahil Gibran summarized when he said that "Much of your pain is self-chosen. It is the bitter potion by which the physician within you heals your sick self. Therefore trust the physician and drink his remedy in silence and tranquility: for his hand though heavy and hard, is guided by the tender hand of The unseen ...." See Psalms 94:19

A good example of self-talk that has no vestige of egotism but which engenders self-esteem that recognizes human limitations before the true God is found at Philippians 4:13.

I once had a sickness that nearly took my life. It made me pass excrement 35 times within 3 days even while taking recommended medication by my physician. On the third night, I was passing excrement when a surge of unexpected dizziness engulfed my whole body within seconds. Is it a drug reaction? No, I was on a doctor's prescription which could even be purchased over-the-counter. What was it? I do not know [this helps to explain that I am not all-knowing]. What did I do with the remaining specters of my consciousness at that moment? I engage in an unuttered prayer to the only true God Jehovah. See Romans 8:26.27. What was the result? I began to regain my conscious balance gradually until I fell asleep and did not wake up until the next morning. Have you seen what positive auto-suggestion can do?

An unenlightened person may find it difficult to decipher which part of the experience forms positive auto-suggestion. The positive auto-suggestion in the experience is the unuttered prayer. Faithless scientists say that prayer is a psychological crunch and some rambling philosophers say that religion is the opium of the masses. This statement may be true of false religions but is not true of true religion. If you cannot comprehend the import of the personal story I just narrated, can you imagine what it would look like to be found dead stark naked while defecating?

An enlightened environment might carry out an autopsy to find out the cause, but would a religious environment enamored with superstitious belief do so? You probably already know that it might be viewed as a just world cause -the widespread false belief that the world is essentially fair so that the good are rewarded and the bad punished. One consequence of this belief is that people

who suffer misfortunes are assumed to deserve their fate.
That was why Andre Gide wrote that "The belief that becomes true for me... is that which allows me the best use of my strength, the best means of putting my virtues into action."

True religious belief enables its devotees to put their "virtues into action", the reverse is the case with most religious beliefs -that produces in its devotees "actions" that are the very opposite of godly devotion See Titus 1:16.
"Know what you believe."-Rudy Giuliani advised. Why? Is belief not an unquestioned acceptance of an idea in faith? That is a well-questioned description of false belief or credulity.
True belief that becomes faith is defined in the Holy Bible at Hebrews 11:1.
"Nothing holds more power over the body than belief."- Deepak Chopra.

True religious belief allows its adherents to question their beliefs, to research or investigate them so that they can appreciate what they possess. See Acts 17:11.

Therefore, be careful in what you accept personally into your belief system through your self-talk or knowledge assimilation, because whether it is negative or positive, it propels you into action. And this action can be internal action or external action. External actions are the ones you act out but internal actions are propelled by your beliefs which govern your thoughts, emotions, and immune system.

Norman Cousins concurred with this same line of thought when he said that " purpose and determination are not merely a mental state. They have electrochemical connections that affect the immune system."

The only difference between negative and positive religious beliefs in its adherents is the effect of their actions on the name of the deity whom they profess to serve. Malachi 3:16-18; Acts 15:14.

Those who become staunch in false beliefs do not question it. Why is this so?
It is because "We would rather be ruined than changed. We would rather die in our dread than climb the cross of the moment. And let our illusions die."- W.H. Auden

Can one who is overreached by his "illusions" overcome it?
The truth is that "Human beings can alter their lives by altering their attitudes of mind."-Dr. William James, the father of American psychology.
When a person's "attitude of mind" is "altered" to the extent that the individual achieves peace of mind, that is what I call…

INTERNAL EQUILIBRIUM
How can a person achieve internal equilibrium -which is another name for peace of mind?
Psychologist Bob Phillips provides he answer when he wrote that "To make positive
changes in your life you must begin by doing something different -especially if what you are doing presently is not bringing happiness."

Peace of mind is difficult to sustain in a mind that is negative and that radiates negative actions. See Isaiah 48:22; 57:20 21.
Why is this so? You can only achieve peace of mind by thinking positive thoughts which produce positive actions.
"He who cannot change the very fabric of his thoughts will never

be able to change reality." - Anwar El Sadat, In Search of Reality.

That is the true "reality". A person who cannot be able to change the very fabric of his thoughts cannot achieve peace of mind. How can this change come about? The most widely distributed book in the world, the Holy Bible at Hebrews 4:12 says that "the word of God is full of living power. It is sharper than the sharpest knife for cutting deep into our innermost thoughts and desires. It exposes us for what we are."-New living Translation.

When you read and apply what you are learning from the Bible the result would be internal equilibrium if coupled with adherence to true religious beliefs and godly devotion. See Psalms 1:1-3; 1Timothy 6:6. Religious beliefs and teachings that I received from Jehovah's Witnesses helped me to gain peace of mind. Despite battling with the worst mental illness called schizophrenia, an illness that turns the mind of its possessor into a universal battlefield. See Neurochemical Factor in chapter three –

The story of my madness for more on this.
How did I achieve lasting peace of mind? I've learned that God's Kingdom -a heavenly government in the hand of Jesus Christ and his 144,000 co-rulers will soon rule over the Earth. See Daniel 2:44; 7:13,14; Revelation 5:9,10; 14:1-3.
That it will remove every sort of sickness and disorders among other things. See Isaiah 33:24. It gives me peace of mind beyond knowing that my health challenge although permanent from a human viewpoint is temporary in the eyes of my God Jehovah. See 2 Corinthians 4:18

Vaclav Havel clarified the benefits of having a better conscience when he said, "In all circumstances try to be decent, just, tolerant and understanding; and at the same time try to resist corruption and deception. In other words, I must do my utmost to act in harmony with my conscience and my better self."

After acquiring the religious beliefs of Jehovah's witnesses, I have become more "decent, just [and] tolerant" with others. Previously before I learned the religious beliefs of Jehovah's Witnesses, I used to disregard the proddings of my "conscience" but now I "act in harmony with my conscience" and as a result, my "better self" or my inner person is at peace with itself. See Romans 2:15.

Acting according to the proddings of positive thought will bring one into an internal equilibrium or peace with oneself- and into an external equilibrium - peace with God and with fellow man. For years many have thought that the best way to stop anger in oneself or another person is by use of angry words. The truth is that anger elicits more anger. See Proverbs 15:1.

When a neuron is stimulated, it runs or travels to a highway called an axon to deliver the message to another neuron. This travel takes place within milliseconds and when a neuron delivers its message, it can elicit the travel of other neurons that are not even in the same category within milliseconds.

Epictetus wrote that "Whenever you are angry, be assured that it is not a present evil, but that you have increased the habit."
In their book entitled: "Pressure Point", psychologists Jay Oliver Ph.D. and H.Norman Wright clarified some reasons why women's attitude seems incomprehensible at times. Under the subheading "Why women get angry", they listed the following as factors that lead them into anger.
(1) when I'm not taking care of
(2) when I sin
(3) Dealing with children

(4) Unfair comparison
(5) Abandonment
(6) Unrealistic expectations
(7) Stress, feeling sorry for myself
(8) Disrespect, people talking behind my back
(9) Discrimination because I'm a woman
(10) Not dealing with previous anger
(11) Over commitment, tired and worn out
(12) Being a people-pleaser
(13) Lack of affection from a spouse
(14) Feeling insecure around people
(15) Selfish demand and not enough quiet time for myself
(16) Entitlement of men, having to wait.
(17) Getting older, PMS (post menstrual syndrome)
(18) When I see I've gained weight
(19) When I've been embarrassed or laughed at
(20) Teenagers and in-laws not having my feelings valued
(21) When I've been used or betrayed.

The authors went further to explain that the root causes of women's anger are fear, frustration, and hurt.
To women who have children, the "pressure" seems to be more unbearable when their children's emotional expression seems unfathomable.

"Remember this rule about child behavior: focus on the course of the behaviors, not the behaviors themselves." Wrote Dr. Blaise Ryan of Child Brain Health Inc. Education research institute and parents learning club.com.
He further advised parents to do this: "Use these three happy child parenting questions to uncover the cause of your child's behaviors... (1) Does my child have a legitimate unmet need? Such as nutrition, water, attention, closeness, sense of belonging,

respect, rest, affection, exercise, stimulation, learning, security, autonomy, socializing, etc.
(2) Does my child need more information? Take another look at your child's unique rhythm for learning. Perhaps he/she may be too young to understand or remember a rule or perhaps more explanation and repetition is needed. (3) Does my child have an accumulation of unprocessed physical or emotional pain or stress? Your child may be experiencing strong emotions, he/she may be scared, angry or resentful, disappointed, hurt, insecure, etc. Stress can be caused by feelings of isolation, criticism, and experiences that are too hard to express - like violence on TV or news. For more tips about kids visit www.parentlearningclub.com and www.jw.org. See Proverbs 22:6.

A child expert speaking against the practice of overloading children with information stated that it is "During the cold spikes of inappropriate pressure into the malleable heart of a child's learning may seriously distort the unfolding of both intellect and motivation. This self-serving intellectual assault, increasingly condemned by teachers who see its warped products, reflects a more general ignorance of the growing brain... Explaining things to children won't do their job; they must have the chance to experience wonder, experiment, and act it out for themselves. It is this process throughout life that enables the growth of intelligence"

In as much as it is true that children need intellectual learning, it must be noted that the most important learning during the formative stages of their life is spiritual, emotional, and social-based learning.

Simon A. Grolnick, writing in the work and Play of Winnicott says that "Play in childhood and throughout the life cycle helps to relieve the tension of living, helps define... the boundaries between ourselves and others, helps give us a sense of our own personal and bodily being. Playing provides drive satisfaction... Winnicott repeatedly stressed that when playing becomes too drive-infested and excited it loses its creative growth building capacity and begins to move towards loss of control or a fetishistic rigidity... Civilizations demands for controlled, socialized behavior gradually, and sometimes insidiously, supersedes the psychosomatic and aesthetic pleasures of open system play."

Therefore, if you are a parent, realize that your child needs a fuller sense of [their] own personal and bodily being, and playing enables them to achieve it.
While it is your responsibility to protect them, providing them opportunities for a reasonable open system play can enable them to experience wonder, experiment and act life out for themselves. Such opportunities have a beneficial effect. It "enables the growth of intelligence -throughout life."
Granted, it is not easy to accomplish this task of child-rearing. It calls for tenacity, maturity - both emotionally and physically and spiritually. Such obligation to our offspring also brings benefits to the parents both immediately and in the later years.

Lin Yutang in his work The Pleasure of a Non-Conformist wrote that "we all have obligations and duties towards our fellow men. But it does seem curious enough that in modern, neurotic society, men's energies are consumed in making a living, and rarely in living itself. It takes a lot of courage for a man to declare with clarity and simplicity that the purpose of lifee is to enjoy it."

In this specialty of intelligence called intrapersonal [individual]

intelligence, we have uncovered how an individual could correlate all the vestiges of his being to achieve an outcome that typifies a good knowledge of self. The way an individual perceives and talks to himself has a greater effect on who he finally becomes consistently.
"For as he thinks within himself, so he is."-Proverbs 23:7-New American Standard Version

This is why effort is needed to see to it that a person leverages organized positive thinking so that his behavior would bring positive benefits to him and others.
When angry, positive self-talk can help you or those who are angry against you.
Dalai Lama uttered a statement that is in this stream of thought when he said that "The way to change other's minds is with affection and not anger."
This is true because anger produces anger when used to counteract a contention. See Proverbs 15:18.
We have also come to know that positive thinking and positive auto-suggestions also produce positive actions but negative thinking and negative auto-suggestions produce
negative actions. See Proverbs 17:14.

The purpose of mastering intrapersonal intelligence is to enable a person to have peace of mind or internal equilibrium. Can a person be happy without having peace of mind? Yes.
How can it be? Peace of mind or internal equilibrium can only be possessed by those who have intrinsic personal peace with the true God Jehovah. It is a lasting internal state enjoyed by the individual possessor as long as the processor is in a permanent spiritual relationship with God. It is unknown to those who do not have a permanent relationship with God. For the avoidance of doubt, the personal peace of mind that I mean is that

which is permanent with God and cannot be extinguished. This spiritual peace of mind is different from secular peace of mind. Secular peace of mind is transient while spiritual
peace of mind is permanent. As long as a person remains devoted to God, nothing can take the peace of mind away. But a secular peace of mind is fleeting- it is produced by happiness. Happiness is a fleeting emotion that can be experienced by any free will intelligent creature, whether the person does good or bad. If you doubt my conclusion that happiness is a fleeting emotion, follow me to experiment with the truthfulness of my conclusions by walking through "The Happy Door" experienced by Mildred Cram who said that "There is no exact definition of the word happiness. Happy people are happy for all sorts of reasons. The key is not wealth or physical well-being, since we find beggars, invalids, and so-called failures that are extremely happy [at times].

Being happy is a sort of an unexpected dividend. But staying happy is an accomplishment. A triumph of soul and character. It is not selfish to strive for it. It is indeed our duty. Being unhappy is like an infectious disease; it causes people to shrink away from the sufferer. He soon finds himself alone, miserable, and embittered. There is, however, a cure so simple as to seem at first glance, ridiculous: if you don't feel happy, pretend to be. It works. Before long you will find that instead of repelling people, you attract them. You discover how deeply rewarding it is to be the center of wild cycles of Goodwill. Then the make-believe becomes a reality. You possess the secret of peace of mind and can forget yourself in being of service to others. Being happy, once it is realized as a duty and established as a habit, opens doors into unimaginable gardens thronged with grateful friends."
Who among mankind has not felt "embittered" since birth? Does a person who serves others not experience ill- will sometimes

even while in the act of service? If this is not true there won't be workers who are disgruntled because of improper motivation.

Granted, having a good relationship with friends engenders a peaceful state of mind in us, but are we always with our friends? Even while enjoying secular peace of mind with our friends, do they always speak words that perfectly please our senses? If you remember any of such moments with your true friends that made you feel embittered, should you discard them because of their thoughtless remarks?

Knowing that true friends are essential in managing life complexities -according to interpersonal intelligence, it will be encouraging to pay attention to Marcus Aurelius who said that "If you are distressed by anything external the pain is not due to the thing itself but to your estimate of it, and this you have the power to revoke at any moment."

It is a person who knows the secrets of mind that can always become happy and have the ability to stop or avoid anything that prevents or hinders his peace of mind. The secrets of peace of mind are twofold. External and internal. The external is to have peace with your fellow man. Have many but few close friends. What "if you are distressed by the external"? You can lessen your "estimate" of external "pain". If you cannot be able to lessen your estimate of the external cause of pain, you can "revoke" it all together and focus on the internal.
The internal is to be at peace with God and you will be at peace with yourself.
"Life without true Godly devotion is inane and devoid of genuine satisfaction and meaning."- Pious Enwereonu. See Ecclesiastes 12:13. Happiness is a step toward peace of mind and the first step

to enduring happiness is assimilating and practicing true spirituality. Keep cultivating your intrapersonal intelligence for it is the center point of other specialties of intelligence.

Chuck Gallozzi said that "We have an innate desire to endlessly learn, grow and develop. We want to become more than what we already are. Once we yield to this inclination for continuous and neverending improvement, we lead a life of endless accomplishment and satisfaction."

INCORPOREAL [INTANGIBLE] INTELLIGENCE

F. Scott Fitzgerald wrote that "The test of a first-rate intelligence is the ability to hold two opposed ideas in the mind at the same time, and still retain the ability to function."

CHAPTER THREE

THE STORY OF MY MADNESS: MENTAL ILLNESS

[SCHIZOPHRENIA]

What is madness? Simply put madness is disorderliness of the mind. It is also called insanity. There are different types of mental illness. The type of mental illness that I suffer from is called schizophrenia. What is schizophrenia? It is a long-term mental disorder of a type involving a breakdown in the relation between thoughts, emotion, and behavior, leading to faulty perception, inappropriate actions, and feelings, withdrawal from reality and personal relationships into fantasy and delusions, and a sense of mental fragmentation.

In short, it is a mental disorder that affects a person's ability to think, feel and behave clearly.

There are different types of schizophrenia; they are paranoid schizophrenia, hebephrenic, schizophrenia, catatonic schizophrenia, undifferentiated schizophrenia, residual schizophrenia, simple schizophrenia, and unspecified schizophrenia.

In this book, I will be using schizophrenia interchangeably with madness.

Psychiatric researchers believe that many factors are responsible for schizophrenia {madness]

(1) Genetic factor. According to researchers, the frequency of schizophrenia in the general population is less than 1%. But being related to someone with schizophrenia greatly increases your risk of developing schizophrenia to 10%. If both parents have it, your risk is 36%.

How this factor affected me: My younger sister developed schizophrenia before me. I was also a caregiver to her for many years while holding a stressful job.

(2) Developmental theory: This theory asserts that something went wrong during the developmental stages of the infant's brain. The following are risk factors for schizophrenia-related critical periods in fetal development, such as :
(A) Children whose mothers experienced famine during the first trimester are more likely to develop schizophrenia.
(B) Schizophrenia is more common in winter and spring births.
(C) Pregnancy and birth complications increase the risk of developing schizophrenia.
How this factors affected me: My mother told me that she experienced ill health when I was a toddler. That illness made her breastfeed me with only one side of her breast.

(3) Neurochemical theory: Some scientists believe that schizophrenia is caused by irregularities in the chemicals of the brain that allow themselves to communicate with each other. "The scientific truth is that all activities in the body are powered by electrical impulses generated in relevant structures. The brain is the main power House of this electrical activity.

This involves the generation of what is known as ACTION POTENTIAL that is propagated along the nerves and on getting to the end of that particular nerve, this impulse is passed to the next nerve by the aid of chemicals known as NEUROTRANSMITTERS. These chemicals are found at junctions between nerves known as SYNAPSES. The ones of interest to us here are DOPAMINE, GLUTAMATE, and SEROTONIN."-Dr. Emmanuel Enabulele.

How this factor affected me: During the illness, my critical mind overwhelmed me with a lot of chattering thoughts. I would feel as though millions of individuals are talking to me simultaneously. One would say "I am Jesus Christ". Another I will say "no I am Barack Obama". Another would say "I am Pious Enwereonu". "Don't believe everything you hear-even in your mind." -Daniel G. Amen, MD Clinical Neuroscientist, Psychiatrist, and Specialist in ADD.

The irregularities of chemical connections in the brain of schizophrenics lead to behaviors that are observed as abnormal. That is why "Everyone can remember something and laugh, but people that are not normal don't just laugh because they remember something. They laugh because they hear voices talking to them. It is due to disruption in the neuronal cells in the brain which is sending abnormal information." -Dr. Kehinde Shodimu, consultant psychiatrist Lagos University Teaching Hospital

(4) Stress Theory: It is a known scientific fact that psychological stress has physiological effects and is implicated in contributing to psychiatric disorders.

How this factor affected me: Before my first experience of madness in 2013, I was highly stressed at work. I was performing the job of four men at the same time. Did you complain? Of course but was not given a fair hearing at mid-level management.

Until I wrote an article in the Dawn Newspaper of Monday 12th November -Sunday 24th November 2012, entitled "Effective Management As Precursor To Effective Motivation.

In the article, I stated among other things: "Humans get tired after dissipation of energy no matter their age. The natural solution is rest. This natural solution does not engender indolence but a revitalization of vital biological processes for the effective output called productivity or service delivery. Achieving productivity with defiance to this natural solution leads to boredom, lack of job satisfaction, and a gradual decline in unleashing latent potentials of self-motivated organizational 'volunteers' whose phantasmagoric(vision) goal is to make a difference in the sands of time."

Granted, some level of stress is required to be productive in the workplace. In fact, " work is not an ethical Duty imposed upon us from without by a misguided and outmoded puritan morality. It is a manifestation of man's desire that the days of his life shall have significance."-Harold W. Dodds.

However, it is a scientific fact that excessive stress leads to mental maladies.
Psychologist Bob Phillips wrote that "The human body cannot withstand stress and pressure for an extended period without some form of negative response."

The stress I endured owing to such overwork started around April 2012 and continued in September 2013- when I developed madness.
"It is well-known that psychological experience - for example, battle stress -can profoundly affect the chemical, hormonal, and physiological functioning of the body. In psychiatric illness, a

psychological factor in a vulnerable person."- Drs Wender and Klein, In their book: Mind, Mood and medicine.

(5) Spiritual Theory: For ages, there has been a common belief among the credulously religious that mental illness is solely a spiritual problem. This belief even crept into the medical world in the medieval periods.

"When hospitals should have been put in place, psychiatric units were not given priority because people believed it was a spiritual and family matter."-Dr. Kehinde Shodimu, a consultant psychiatrist, Lagos State University Teaching Hospital.

Religious people who believe that mental illness is spiritual leveraged their belief from some biblical accounts that narrated how Jesus healed demons possessed men and women. One typical account that inexorably pointed to spiritual factors to mental illness [schizophrenia], is the account of the Bible book of Luke 8:26-39. It is noteworthy that verse 27 mentioned that the demon-possessed man had not worn clothing, stayed among tombs or isolated places, is violent-according to verses 29, and became "clothed" and in his right [sound] mind after Jesus Christ cured him.

Leveraging from other theories, the reader would understand that spiritual theory is a factor but not the rule. I'm a minister of God. And not a medical doctor but a sufferer of schizophrenia and as such, I have a say on both dichotomies of spiritual or medical causes and solutions to mental illness.
"Winners of the Nobel prize are not more competent about God and religion and life after death than other people." -Nobel laureate, Vladimir Prelog.

To give you my experience and opinion on the two dichotomies, I will recreate the conversation that I had with one of my female religiously inclined colleagues during my relapse in mental illness in 2018. For the sake of ensuring her right to privacy, I will call her the name Tabitha. I sent the following message on WhatsApp to people on the list, including Tabitha: "What is the difference between craziness and madness?

Tabitha: My brother, happy new month please kindly come to our church for deliverance. The Bible makes us understand that because of lack of knowledge my people perish. I'm not saying that you should go to Babalawo [native doctor] or any of such. But I said come to church to receive your healing and the deep things that you don't know.

Author: What are those deep things that I don't know. Tell me I'm listening.

Tabitha: Oh you've learned all. The word of God is always new and fresh. Through it, you will receive your healing I promise you.

Author: I have not known all I need to know in life. But I have known much to know that church is the epicenter of both physical and spiritual madness. I have attended ten churches before I became a Jehovah's witness. My younger sister and one of my younger brothers have the same psychiatric illness that I'm battling with. Do you know that my parents who are not Jehovah's witnesses carried my younger siblings for crazy deliverance from one church to another but instead of healing them, their conditions became worse?

Tabitha: Let me tell you, take it or you leave it. The church is the solution. Going to different churches does not mean that the church cannot cure it. The God I'm serving, the God of untouchable will heal you in Jesus' name. Do you call it crazy Deliverance? May God Have Mercy on you, my brother.

Author: In the medieval period, it was believed that madness is caused by demons but in our modern enlightened world it is now firmly believed that it is a medical problem. So there are two dichotomous beliefs now. The religious world says it is spiritually caused while the scientific world says it is medical. Since one who wears the shoe knows where it pinches. I'm in a better position to say which dichotomy won in the debate. My answer is no Victor, no vanquished. So craziness is when a dog barks at you and you barks back without knowing fully why it barked. While madness is when the dog bites you and you bite it back without knowing fully that a barking dog can bite.

Tabitha: Please my brother remember that you are not the only one that has the problem.

Author: That is true. So how many people have all the churches in the world cured of their madness? The problem is a dilemma. It is partly spiritual and partly physical. So if you think that you can only use the spiritual to cure the physical you are making a mistake. This is the reason why there are so many mad persons walking around the earth, the church is seeing them but looking the other way despite claims of miracle-working power — Matthew 7:21-23.

So from the foregoing and with authority that I have by being an author of this intellectual work on both corporeal and incorporeal intelligence, I can say with a degree of certainty that craziness is corporeal why madness is incorporeal. In other words, craziness

is medical why madness is spiritual. Craziness is graduation into madness. So among craziness and madness which is synonymous with schizophrenia. Schizophrenia subsumes both. To prevent schizophrenia, prevent the condition that causes craziness.
What is the solution to schizophrenia? There is no permanent solution now. But there are palliatives. What are they? Psychiatric drugs and prayers.

Myopic people who have half-baked knowledge of the facts with religious alacrity postulate that it is only prayer that can solve the dilemma. I disagree. As a sufferer, I can vouch that the effect of prayers on schizophrenia is inner peace of mind and tranquility while the drugs reduce the symptoms and help one to gain perspective.

Conclusively, a mad person is mentally confused during the period of madness. He or she does not know what he or she is thinking throughout madness while a crazy person sometimes unintentionally goes into a lucid period. How did I come to know all of this?
You might ask? You probably already know that uneasiness lies in the head that wears the crown? I live on the knife-edge between genius and insanity. If you doubt the veracity of my verbiages — you can search the online search engines to ascertain whether there has been a sufferer of schizophrenia that produced works of intellectual excellence in their lucid period.

The reader can note the effect of religious belief on Tabitha's insistence that the author should go to her church and receive a cure for his mental illness. Had it been the author is
not a minister of God, and having seen how his parents got their hands burnt in connection with the futile church healing of his younger siblings, he would have been another victim of spiritual

healing deception.

POSITIVE SYMPTOMS OF SCHIZOPHRENIA:
(1) Hallucinations - hearing or seeing or feeling something that is not there. It affects any of the five senses - sound. sight, touch, taste, and smell.

(2) Delusions -believes which are not likely to change when presented with conflicting evidence and which can lead to separating real from unreal experiences.

(3) Agitation- increased tension and becoming more irritable.

NEGATIVE SYMPTOMS OF SCHIZOPHRENIA
These are characterized by a lack of functioning.

(1) Lack of drive or initiative- spending a lot of time in bed or lack of ability to take care of personal appearance or care for oneself.

(2) Social withdrawal/ depression — spending a lot of time alone with no desire to see other people.

(3) Apathy — feelings of emptiness and lack of drive to follow through on plans.

(4) Lack of emotional response -lacking normal signs of emotion. Not feeling happy or sad. Reduced facial expressions.

WARNING SIGNS OF SCHIZOPHRENIA RELAPSE:
(1) Sleeping and eating less or refusing to get out of bed.
(2) Inability to concentrate.
(3) Unusual ideas or strange use of words.

(4) Poor personal hygiene.
(5) Social withdrawal.
(6) Lack of interest and motivation in daily activities.

HOW I MANAGE MY MADNESS [SCHIZOPHRENIA]

(1) PSYCHIATRIC DRUGS: I've been on psychiatric drugs since 2013 when I first experienced the illness. I learned that the illness requires being on medication throughout my lifetime. I have been religiously taking my drugs until the Year 2018 when I had a relapse as a result of the fact that I did not take the drugs for about 3 months. Thereafter I learned from experience the previous theoretical knowledge that a schizophrenic patient need not miss his or her drug for a single day. Relapse rates are far higher when patients are nonadherent with their medication, so you should try your very best to take your medication exactly as it has been prescribed.

(2) PRAYER: Enables me to regain inner peace of mind and tranquility. When praying, I endeavor to apply what Jesus Christ taught in the Bible book of Matthew 6:6-8.
A scientist who is not schooled in the discipline of spirituality may doubt the efficacy of prayer on such chronic mental illness as schizophrenia.

Albert Einstein encouraged fellow scientists to be open-minded regarding spiritual matters when he said that "everyone who is seriously involved in the pursuit of science becomes convinced that some spirit is manifest in the laws of the universe, one that is vastly superior to that of man."

My spiritual routine as one of Jehovah's witnesses enables me to maintain a positive mental attitude. What is that mental attitude

that gives me fortitude?
I know that my illness may be permanent in this life, but it is temporary from the viewpoint of my God Jehovah who's an eternal being. See Psalms 90:2

He has established his kingdom-a heavenly government which he handed over to his son Christ Jesus as King. This Kingdom will soon rule over the entire universe [Daniel 7:13,14; Matthew 6:9,10]

"With increased spirituality, people reduce their sense of self and feel a greater sense of oneness and connectedness with the rest of the universe...."-Dan Cohen, Assistant Professor of Religious Studies.

(3)SLEEP: Helps me regain my mental equilibrium. Without adequate sleep, I notice that the symptoms of my illness subsist. Professor Nick Glozier said that "Changes in lifestyle patterns are a contributing factor to these problems but it's evident that disrupted sleep patterns are a major contributor to many types of mental health conditions."

Professor Glozier was correct because I do recall that after I had missed taking my drugs for three months, I performed a special duty one day that lasted the early hours of the next day. And on that day, the relapse which I mentioned previously ensued. Intermittent sleep during an experience of symptoms enables me to regain sanity.

(4)FOOD: Healthy food is required to maintain good mental health. I can remember that before my first experience of the illness in 2013, I had challenges concerning proper nutrition because I decided to experiment with the benefit of eating less food to live below my means.

"A careful physician..., before he attempts to administer a remedy to his patient must investigate not only the malady of the man he wishes to cure but also his habits when in health and his physical constitution."-Cicero.

During one of my hospital visits, I learned from one of my doctors that fasting is a precipitating factor that endangers sound mental health. He said that the brain needs food and fruits to function optimally.

When he mentioned the relevance of food in my condition, I recalled an experience I had one day when I was feeling the symptoms of my illness surging through my senses. I remember that I had not eaten up to that moment. What I did was eat and immediately after I finished eating the symptoms started to recede. When I coupled it with prayer and sleep I achieved relief even though I did not take my drug because it was not the time to take the drug according to the doctor's prescription.

(5) COLD BATH: I believe that water has curative powers that mankind has not yet discovered.

"Since the molecular structure of water is the essence of all life, the man who can control that structure in cellular systems will change the world."- Albert Szent- Gyorgy, Nobel prize winner.

When I am experiencing a resurgence of schizophrenic symptoms, if it is not yet time for me to take my recommended drugs, what I do first is to pray, next thing is to have a cold bath when I'm at home. If I'm not at home I take cold water and use it to wash my head.

What happens when I take a cold water bath? I usually experience a gradual regaining of sanity. After bathing the next thing I do is to sleep.

(5) WORK: Helps me to satisfy the need for connection. Thereby making a contribution for societal peace. It also makes me to feel relevant and my contribution to secular society very significant. Though, I usually find it challenging to work when I experience a schizophrenic episode. So I make it a duty to inform my colleagues about my condition and this enables them to work cooperatively with me. That is why Psychologist Erik Erikson said that "Life doesn't make any sense without interdependence. We need each other and the sooner we learn that, the better for us all."

(6) CAREGIVERS: When I first experienced schizophrenia in 2013, my aunt Ulunna Amuga and my sibling David Enwereonu cared for me during the month of hospitalization. But during my relapse in 2018, my sibling Judith Enwereonu cared for me. I am very grateful for the love and care they showed me.

(7) ADVICE TO CAREGIVERS: Provide ongoing support and encouragement to your relative or friend who's suffering from Schizophrenia. Never feel ashamed of doing so because of stigmatization associated with the illness. See Proverbs 17:17. People living with schizophrenia are like everyone else. They need to know when they are doing things right or wrong. A positive approach may be more helpful and effective in the long term than criticizing your loved one's thoughts and behavior which may be altered by their condition.

ADVICE TO SCHIZOPHRENIA SUFFERERS: Appreciate your caregivers. It doesn't matter whether they are your siblings or not. Remember, they are sacrificing a lot to care for you. Without them caring for you, you might be among the schizophrenics [madpeople] that are roaming the streets naked and eating from refuse dumps. But when you appreciate them, it will give them the motivation to continue to care for you. At times they may talk to you in a manner you do not like, never take that to mean that they are your enemy. They are not, rather they may be overwhelmed by anxiety caring for you. If you are in a job, let your colleagues know about your condition early enough so that there can work cooperatively with you. The first person among your colleague you should inform is your immediate boss or head of the department. The reason for this dissemination of information concerning your condition to your colleagues is that when you experience a schizophrenic episode, they will be in a better position to help you at least keep your job. Never feel ashamed of your condition. It is a terminal illness just like any other terminal illnesses like stroke, diabetes, and cancer.

CHAPTER FOUR

INTUITIVE INTELLIGENCE

This is the ability to automatically attain direct knowledge or cognition without evident rational thought or inference. An individual can subconsciously leverage this ability during extrapolatory thinking.

The medium through which this knowledge is transferred is what I called Abstract- Cosmic-Magnetism. An individual becomes aware of the presence of intuition after dissipative structures finish exacting a temporary pressure or stress to the recipient. "Chance favors the prepared mind."-Louis Pasteur enthused.
Is intuitive intelligence practicable? Yes. To become intuitively intelligent, you need to practice meditation. Ensure that your environment is quiet. Free from noise. So that you can listen to the voices of your mind.

WARNING: If you are having a schizophrenic episode, "Don't believe everything you hear-even from your mind."-Daniel G.Amen MD Clinical Neuroscientist, Psychiatrist, and Specialist in ADD.
So when do I need to listen to my mind and accept my intuition? That is when you are in a lucid period and can think clearly as a result of adherence to your doctor's treatment regimen. Then, you can be able to distinguish between intuition and autosuggestion [see Intrapersonal Intelligence for autosuggestion meaning]

"If you don't have a daily meditation practice [when you are in lucid period] it is difficult to tell the difference between your critical mind and your intuitive mind."-Emily Fletcher advised.

It is impossible to learn through intuition without being in a meditative mode.

At times an intuition can come into you unexpectedly. This happens because "the intuition whispers" according to Emily Fletcher. Why is it hard to hear intuition when the mind is in busy mode?

"The critical mind is always screaming at us. It is very hard to hear your intuition when your critical mind is screaming at you."- Emily Fletcher, an intuition expert stated.

Which part of the brain is the gateway for intuition?

"Your right brain is a piece of you that is in charge of intuition. Is a piece of you that connects to collective intelligence."- Emily Fletcher added.

Abstract-Cosmic-Magnetism is an incorporeal mechanism that enables two or more people to attract thoughts of similar nature from a distance at the same time.

An example of Abstract-Cosmic-Magnetism is when you are thinking about someone, the person shows up in a moment without any prior communication between you and the person. Abstract- Cosmic-Magnetism is the medium through which the intuitive mind connects to collective intelligence. What Emily Fletcher called "collective intelligence" is what I call the Universal Mind.

See chapter five- Abstract Intelligence for the meaning of Universal Mind.

When intuition comes to you, treat it with care by connecting its content with your core values and purpose of existence. If the content of intuition is uneven with your core values or purpose of existence, I advise that you keep it at abeyance without application.

Follow the rules of the "Law of extrapolation" [states that achievement of an outcome is preceded by consistent adaptive actions based on the initially inferred idea-Pious Enwereonu], at this juncture you will be surprised to find that in the long run, you will still achieve the object of your inferred outcome.

This is because even if you took only one action to achieve an inferred idea, there is a corollary effect to that action.
Another person who is aware of that action you took, and who believes that your action is also in tandem with his own beliefs, values, and purpose may act in furtherance to your own, with or without your knowledge.

Intuition is an Incorporeal thought of a free-willed intelligent creature transferred into the mind of another free-willed intelligent creature through a natural process I call Abstract-Cosmic-Magnetism- via the recipient subconscious mind and which is brought into the individual's knowledge by the reticular activating system [The reticular activating system's fundamental role in regulating arousal and sleep-wake transitions... The ascending projections of the reticular activating system enhance the attentive state of the cortex and facilitate conscious perception of sensory stimuli. Source: https://www.sciencedirect.com]
"The greatest gift you can give another is the purity of your attention."-Richard Moss said.

This is true whether it is in face-to-face conversation or otherwise. If you have programmed your subconscious mind with righteous values and purposes scrutinize any intuition with them before implementation or else you might be working against the realization of your initially inferred outcome. Intuitions occur to accentuate the demands of your subconscious mind. This is true notwithstanding whether you unknowingly programmed your subconscious mind with negative extrapolation or positive extrapolation.

Norman Vincent Peale wrote that "The unconscious is a great dynamo, but it is also a computer that has to be properly programmed. If fear thoughts worry thoughts, failure thoughts are channeled into the unconscious, nothing very constructive is going to be sent back. But if a clear purposeful goal is steadfastly held in the conscious mind, the unconscious will eventually accept and begin to supply the conscious mind with plans, ideas, insights [or intuition], and the energies necessary to achieve that goal."

After an individual finishes examining his or her core values and purpose of existence and feels that the intuition is in agreement with them, the person is advised to apply the intuition, because failure to do so, will relegate the individual to mediocrity.

Albert Einstein said that "Insanity is doing the same thing over and over again while expecting different results." Cultivating and sustaining a virtuous life right now is the best preparation for an intuition that will result in not only an intrinsic value balance but a new idea that can catapult one to more successful living.

Dr. Nnamdi Azikiwe advised that you should "Pray that success will not come any faster than you can endure it."
How can one know for sure that he has intuition? It comes at times as a strong idea which you have never thought of.

Patanjali said that "When you are inspired by some great purpose, some extraordinary project, all your thoughts break their bonds, your mind transcends limitations, your consciousness expands in every direction, and you find yourself in a new great world.

Dormant forces, faculties, and talents become alive, and you discover yourself to be a greater person by far than you ever dreamed yourself to be."

A second sign that the idea is intuition is this: You become more knowledgeable in that subject for which you experienced an intuition.

Oliver Wendell Holmes sums it up when he said that "Man's mind stretched to a new idea never goes back to its original dimension." Despite the ramblings of mind over matter proponents, the author's view is this: Intuition takes place between free-willed intelligent creatures while non- free-willed creatures are governed by instinct. Free-willed intelligent creatures communicate through thinking and feeling but non-free-willed creatures communicate through instinct. Man's professed instinct is nothing but his innermost subsumed feelings, and he can detect the similarity between his and another's intuition.

George Moore said that "Our ideas are today and gone tomorrow, whereas our feelings are always with us, and we recognize those who feel like us at once, by sort of instinct."

CHAPTER FIVE

ABSTRACT INTELLIGENCE

This is the ability to stimulate, imagine and understand ideas, concepts, and abstractions by combining them into one synthesis. It is not a professed allegorical criticism or psychical mysticism but an ability to integrate known facts with new ideation to discover an unknown knowledge. Abstract intelligence is a hallmark of integrative thinking [I will write a chapter on this in my future book].

Einstein is an example of one who possesses abstract intelligence. Imagination according to Albert Einstein is greater than knowledge. Why? Because knowledge is limited but imagination encircles the world. While in the act of "imagination" an individual can easily leverage Abstract-Cosmic -Magnetism if such imagination is unencumbered by self- inhibitory extrapolatory catastrophe occasioned by one's negative critical mind or that of another person in the universal mind pool.

"A so-called genius is only a man who because of his great capacity for enthusiasm, steps up the vibrations of his mind until he is enabled to communicate with a source of knowledge not available to him through his faculty of reason alone."-Author Unknown

As long as there is human existence, the ability to imagine remains a continuum. Why?Because it was an endowed ability.

William Shakespeare once wrote, "I have an immortal longing in me."

It is abstract intelligence that enables man to sustain "immortal longings." When the plane of abstract intelligence reaches its climax with "immortal longings" subsisting,
man can "communicate with a source of knowledge not available to him through his faculty of reason alone." At this point, the subconscious mind is open to suggestions from incorporeal external sources outside the individual. Who and what is made up of these outside "sources of knowledge" which I referred to as the Universal Mind?

WHO?
At the apex of the Universal Mind is the source of eternal intelligence, the most invisible supreme sovereign of the universe, and the only true God Jehovah. He endowed the universe with intelligence.

"The universe is set in an Order such that through keen focus and observation humans can predict and determine necessary outcomes." -Mr. Olakunle Soriyan, economist and philosopher.

After observing the intelligence that is replete in the universe, I define universal intelligence thus: Is a consistent cosmic adaptive action that achieves the initially inferred idea of its originator.

Jehovah God is the originator of the universe. He is not an impersonal God, rather he is the greatest personage in the universe.
"For those who have eyes to see and minds accustomed to reflect, in the minutest cells, in the blood, in the whole earth, and throughout the Stella universe..., there is intelligent and conscious direction; in a word there is mind."-British biologist Alfred Russel Wallace, the co-founder of the theory of

evolution.

Isn't it ironic that the co-founder of the theory of evolution believes in the existence of an intelligent mind who is behind the conscious direction of the universe?

The "mind" behind the "conscious direction" of the "universe" is the greatest "intelligent" mind- Psalms 102:25-27; 1Timothy 1:17. As long as the greatest intelligent mind behind the conscious direction of the universe continues to exist, the universe will continue to exist.
Apart from the supreme Sovereign at the apex of the Universal Mind, others exert influence in the universal mind pool. They are called angels. They are messengers of the universal sovereign.
But some rebelled against the rulership of the universal sovereign. See Bible book of Jude 6.
These rebellious angels are now called demons. They are headed by their Master -Satan the devil. These intelligent creatures on the lower plane of the universal mind pool also exert influence on the lower realm. See John 12:31;1 John 5:19; Revelation 12:9.Ephesians 6:12.They are very wicked and they exact an inordinate sadistic influence over those whom they control. Any wonder why there is so much evil and cruelty in the world? See Genesis 6:2,4,5. Just as true the God destroyed the ancient world because of the influence of the dematerialized demonic angels, he has promised to destroy all evildoers of our time. See Psalms 37:9-11

WHAT?
The universe contains an incorporeal faint consciousness. This is what I call the Universal Mind. There is a plane of deep thinking that a person can reach to harness knowledge from the universal mind. As a result of such harnessing, man has been able to

identify some of the governing principles and laws subsumed in the faintly conscious universe.

Deepak Chopra said that "To understand the magical nature of the mind is to acquire awesome power, it is to understand that at any moment of our life we have the power to accomplish anything we want. In the vast ocean of universal Mind, infinite power is contained and is ours on demand."

To fetch some water from "the vast ocean the Universal Mind", you need to understand the magical nature of the mind. To "understand the magical nature of the mind" you need to have near absolute tranquility. That is the tranquility that is devoid of distractions so that your mind can concentrate on a subject that is your purpose of meditation.
Your mind may try to drive you into a different direction when you are trying to go and fetch water from the ocean of universal Mind, but you need to continue to control your mind for it to remain on course. How can you do that? Endeavor to keep the subject matter in front of your journey constantly. Before beginning your mental journey into the ocean of universal Mind, imagine yourself fetching water from the ocean and back into your mind. See yourself in your mind's eye enjoying the benefit of successfully fetching water from the ocean. What exactly can I set as subject matter? The author cannot answer that because he is not in your mind.

Your mind knows its desires and needs. However, the author has this warning for you: Remember the persons that influence the universal Mind pool which we discussed in the preceding WHO? Your choice of desire, need, or want will be dependent on your belief system.

Anton Chekhov once said: "Man is what he believes." Your "beliefs" will guide you. This is irrespective of whether they are positive or negative beliefs. But I would encourage you to cultivate positive beliefs. Why? Because "If you realize how powerful your thoughts are, you would never think negative thoughts." Peace Pilgrim advised.

Thoughts form beliefs. What thoughts are positive? "Whatever things are true, whatever things are of serious concern, whatever things are righteous, whatever things are chaste, whatever things are lovable, whatever things are well spoken of, whatever things are virtuous, and whatever things are praiseworthy, continue considering these things. The things that you learned as well as accepted and heard and saw in connection with me, practice these and the God of peace will be with you."-Philippians 4:8,9; Galatians 5:22,23. New World Translation of the Holy Scriptures.

CONCLUSION

Schizophrenia is the worst type of illness because it is an illness that the sufferer does not know that he or she is ill during the time of the illness. One who is a sufferer can live a healthy life though if he or she could stick to his or her prescription regimen.

Other lifestyle factors that contribute to sound health after experiencing schizophrenia include having adequate night sleep. Having or eating a good meal according to one's means. Attending doctor's visits for a check-up. Relating well with one's caregivers – friends, relatives, and acquaintances.

It is wrong to stigmatize schizophrenia sufferers. Because just like other terminal illnesses such as stroke, cancer, and diabetes schizophrenia is a brain illness. So just as one shows empathy to patients of other terminal illnesses that is how compassion should be shown to those who suffer from schizophrenia.

ABOUT THE BOOK

We are conversant with the sight of mad people who roam the streets, parks, and isolated places. Some are naked while some wear tattered clothing and look unkempt.

The book uncovers what goes on in the mind of a mad person [schizophrenia].
How to live a healthy life after experiencing mental illness [schizophrenia]. And what to do to assist a relative or friend as a caregiver.

ABOUT THE AUTHOR

Pious Enwereonu is a minister of God. He is also a policeman who has worked in various formations and departments such as finance, investigation and is currently in administration at Enugu State Police Headquarters.

He is a researcher and a former writer for The Dawn Newspaper. He has read more than 300 books on personal development, psychology, policing, spirituality, mentorship, finance, and health.

You can reach him at his email address:
enwereonupious402021@gmail.com.

www.ingramcontent.com/pod-product-compliance
Lightning Source LLC
Chambersburg PA
CBHW070123230526
45472CB00004B/1387